# THE PICTURE BOOK OF

# TEACUPS

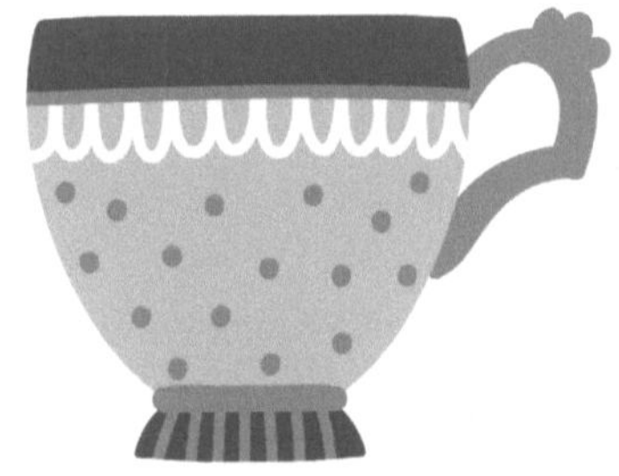

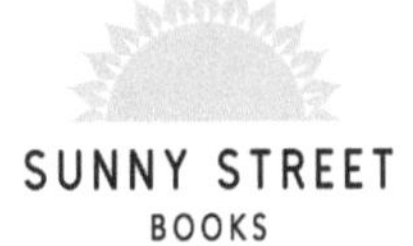

SUNNY STREET
BOOKS

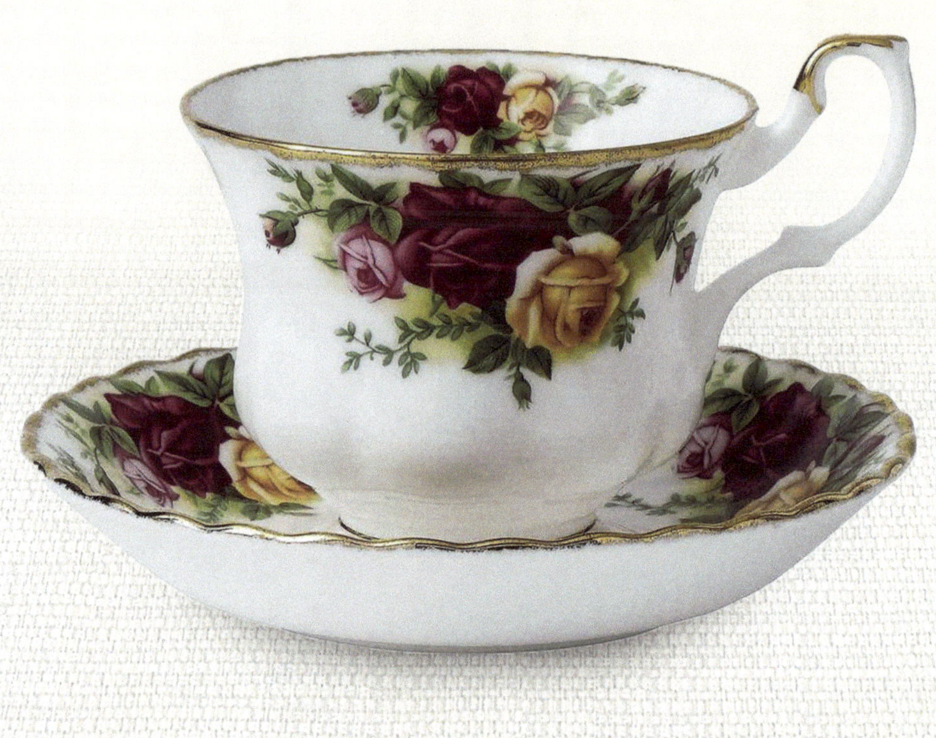

# ROYAL ALBERT
## OLD COUNTRY ROSES

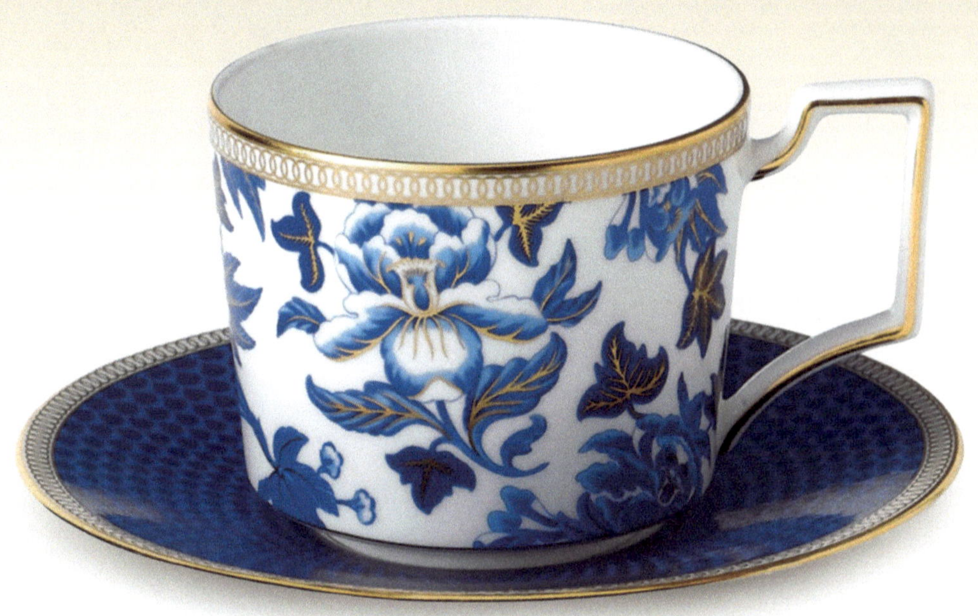

# WEDGWOOD

## HIBISCUS

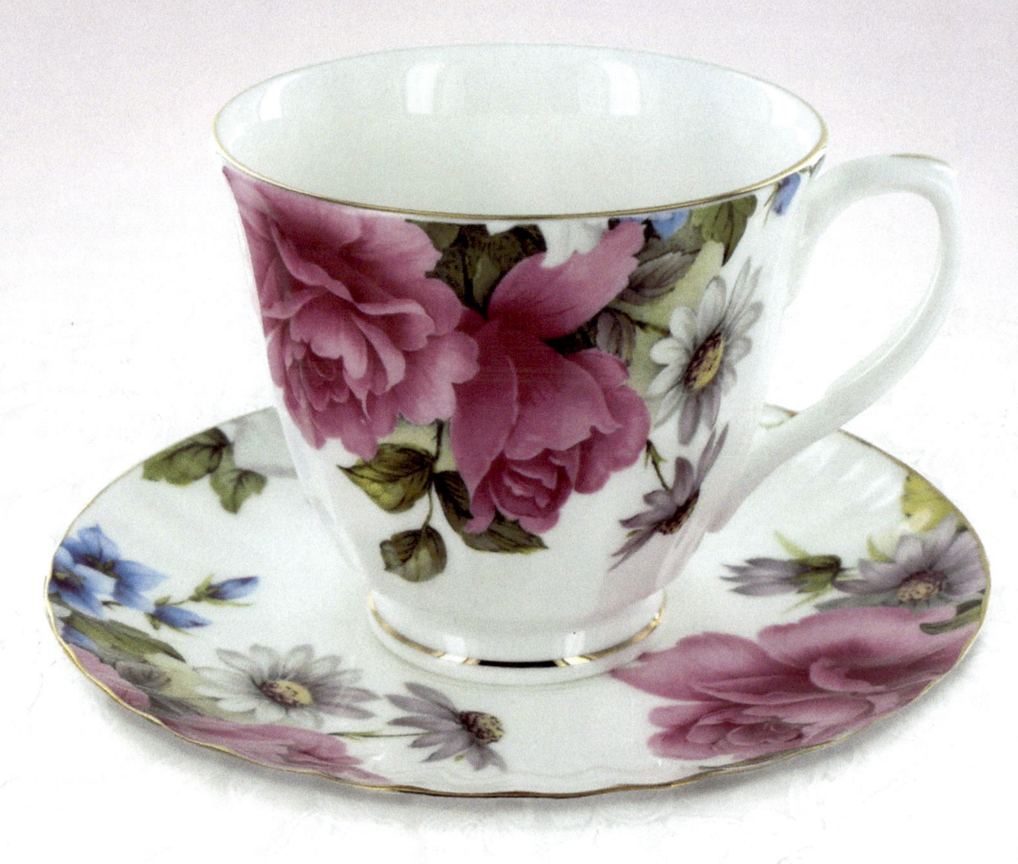

# GRACIE BONE CHINA

## ROSE CHINTZ

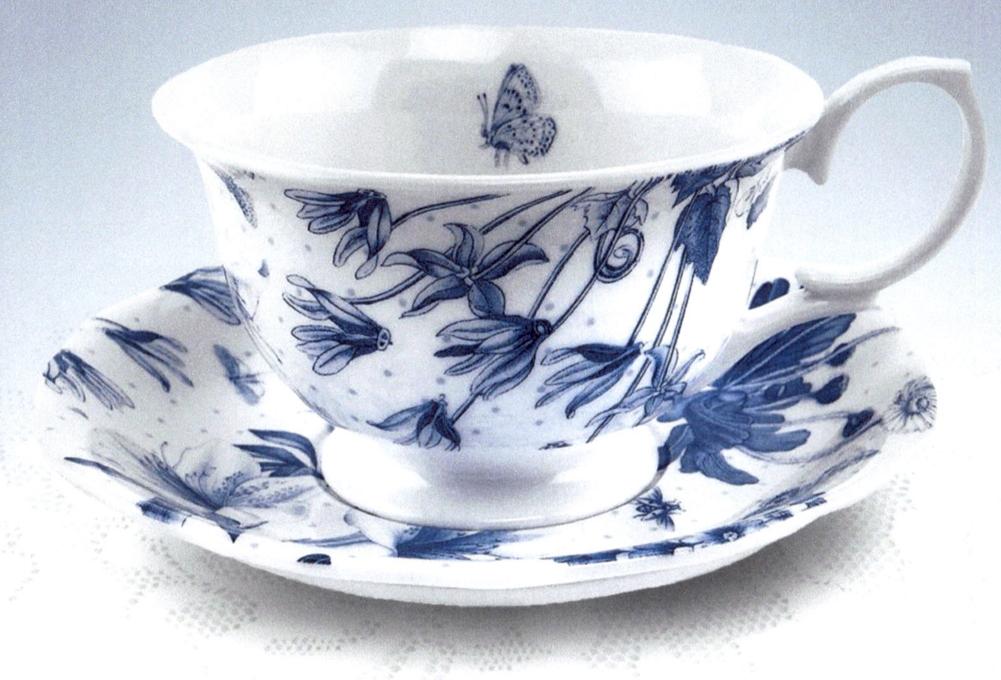


PORTMIERION

BOTANIC BLUE

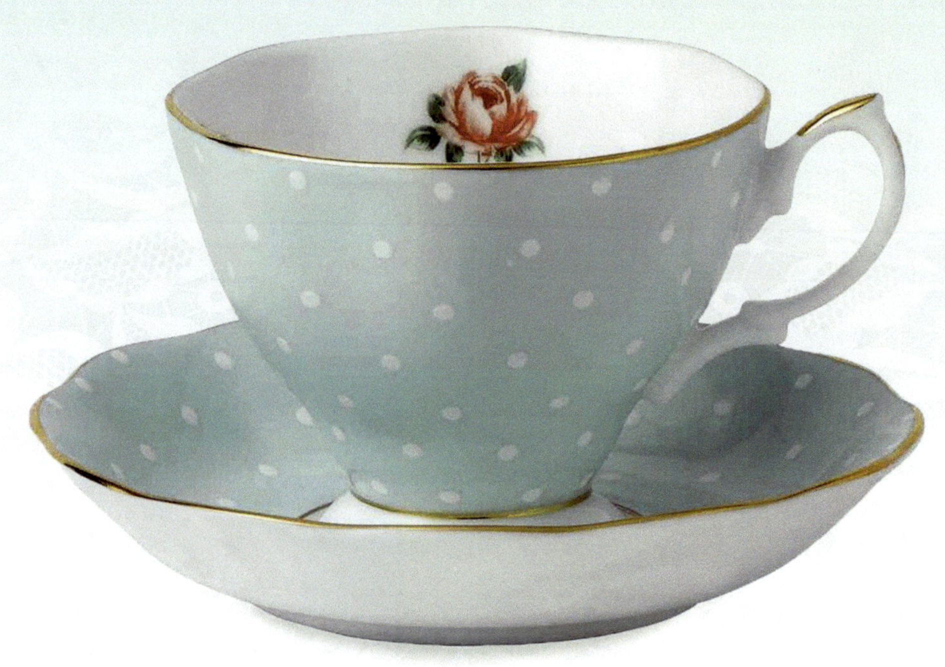

# ROYAL ALBERT

## POLKA ROSE

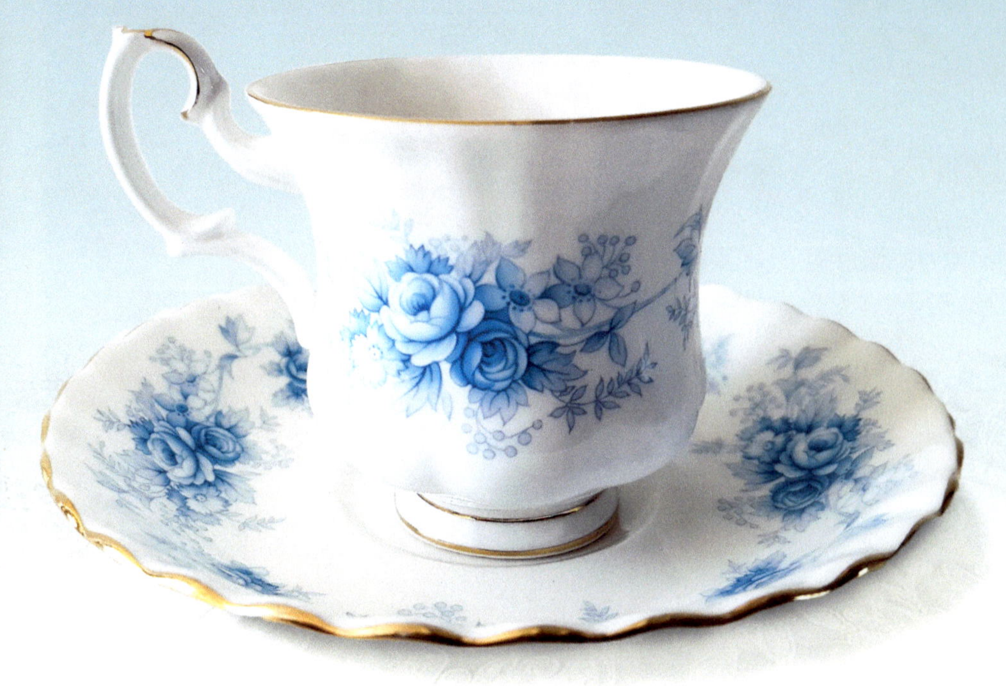

# ROYAL ALBERT
## WINDSOR ROSE

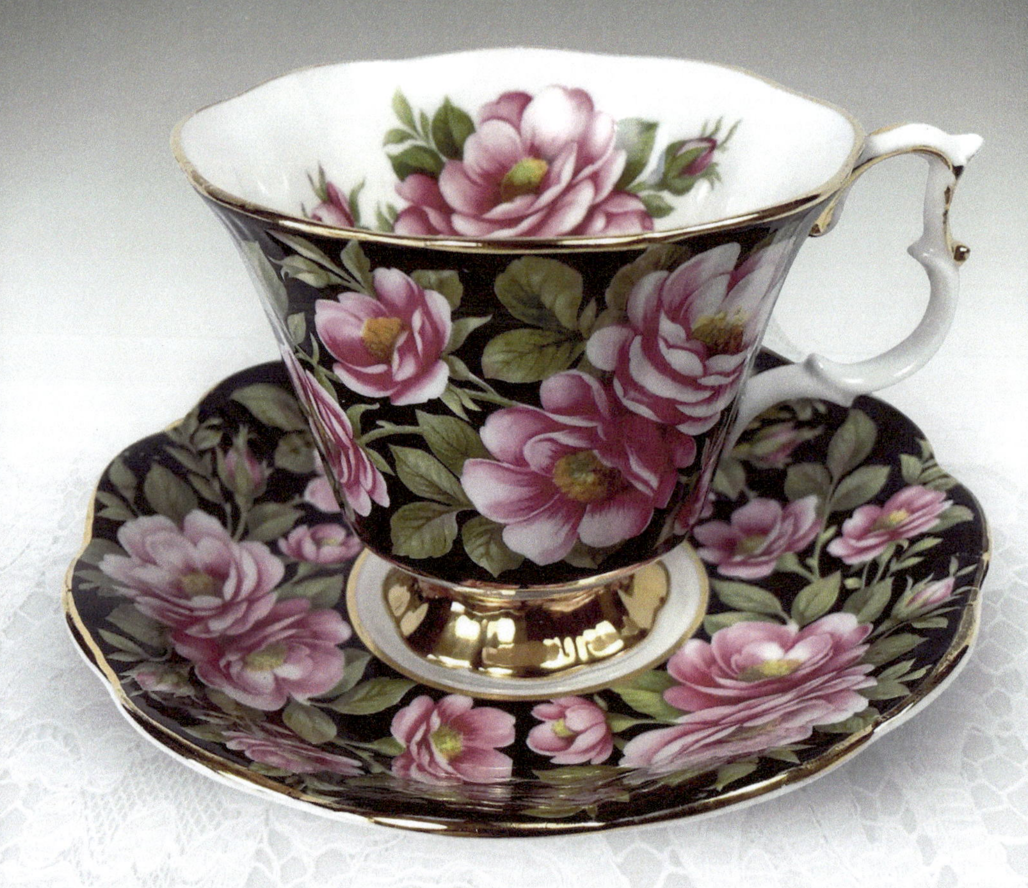

# ROYAL ALBERT
## RAMBLER ROSE CHINTZ

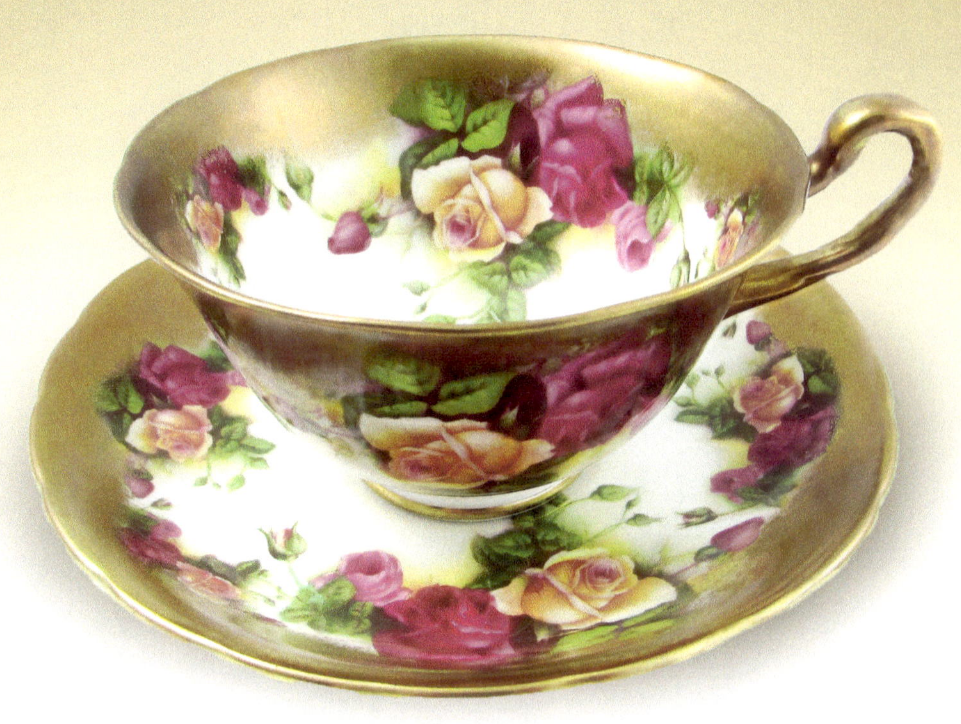

# ROYAL CHELSEA

## GOLDEN ROSE

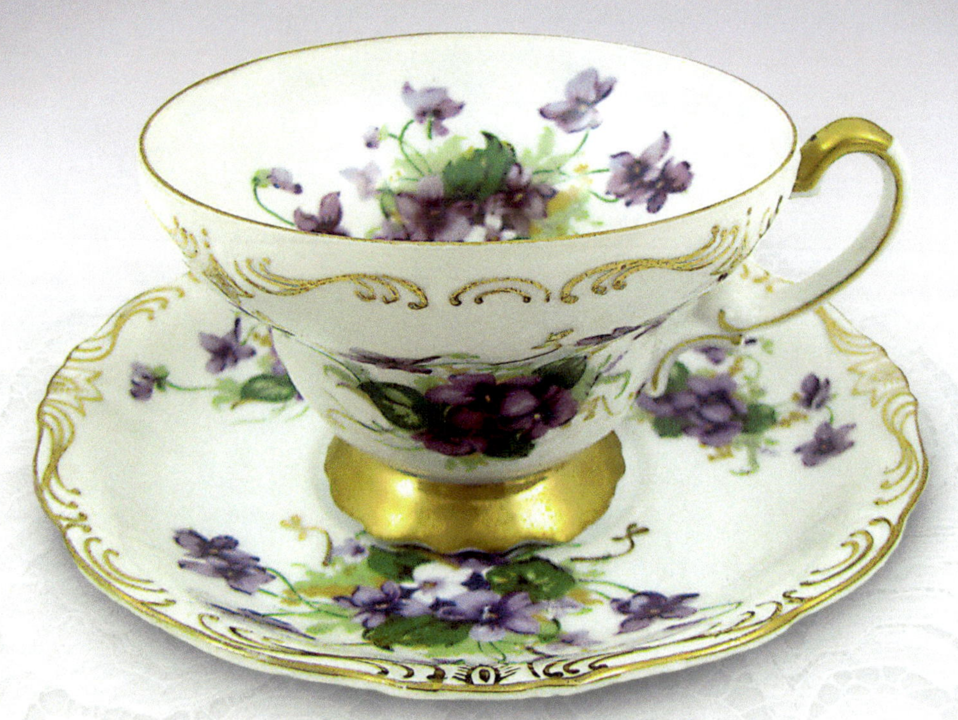

# Norcrest

## Sweet Violets

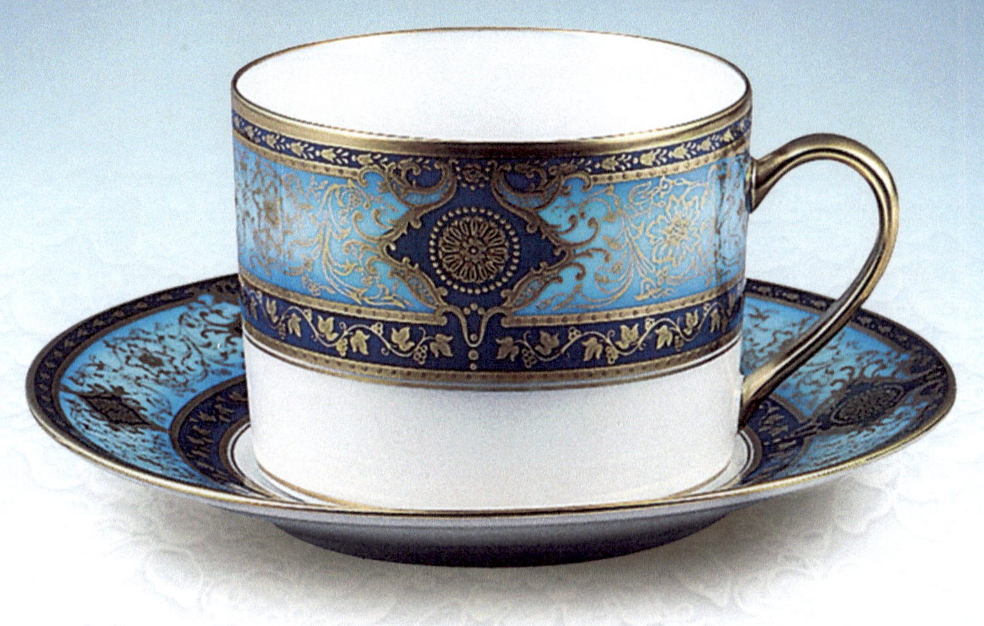

# BERNARDAUD

## GRACE

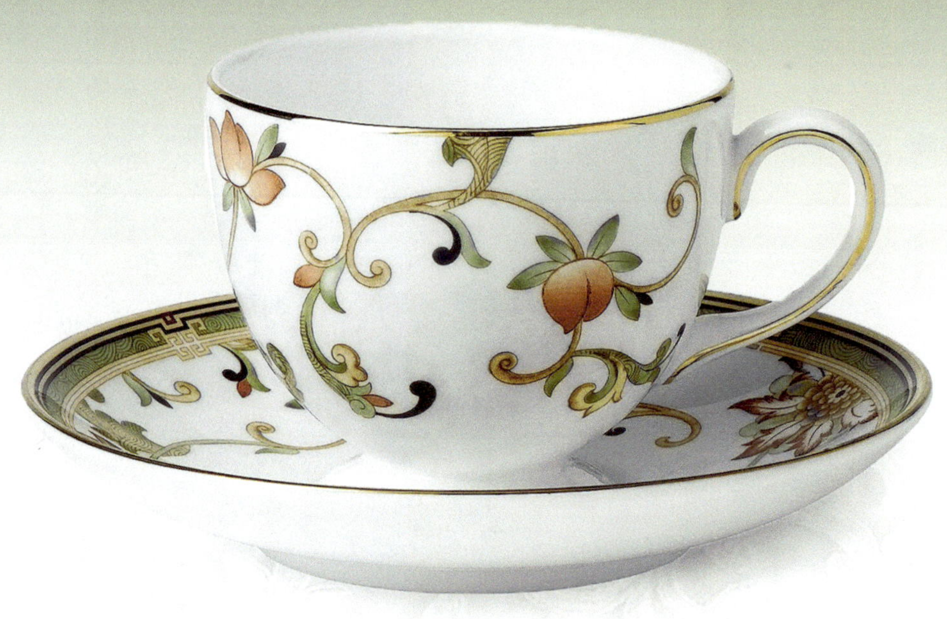

# WEDGEWOOD

## OBERON

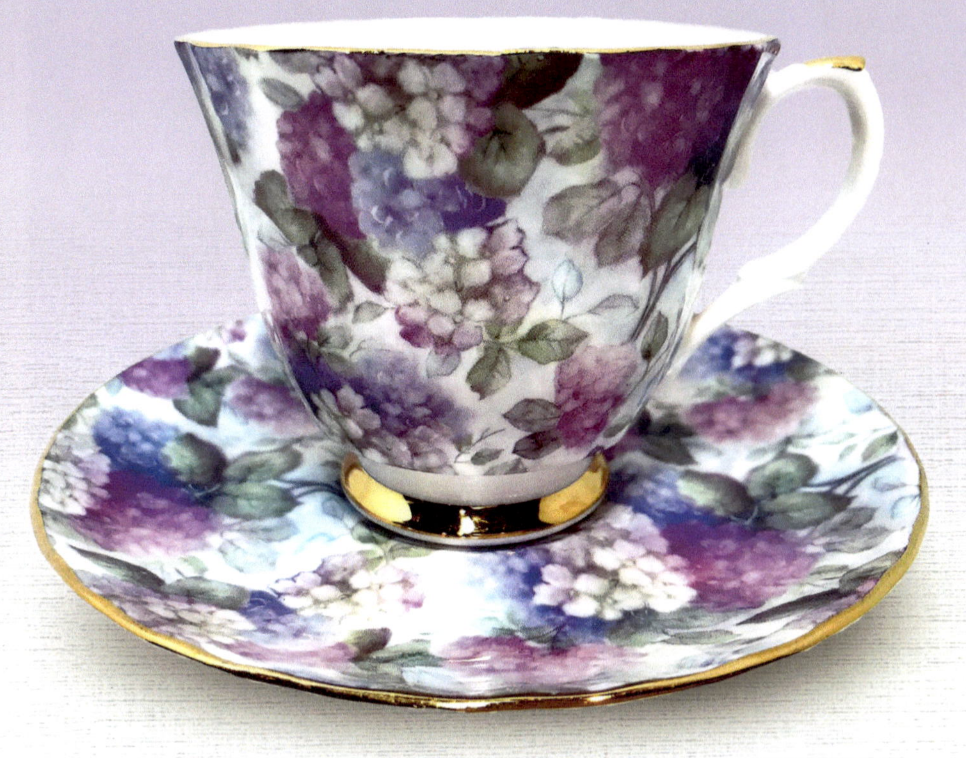

# ROYAL PATRICIAN

## LOVELY LILAC

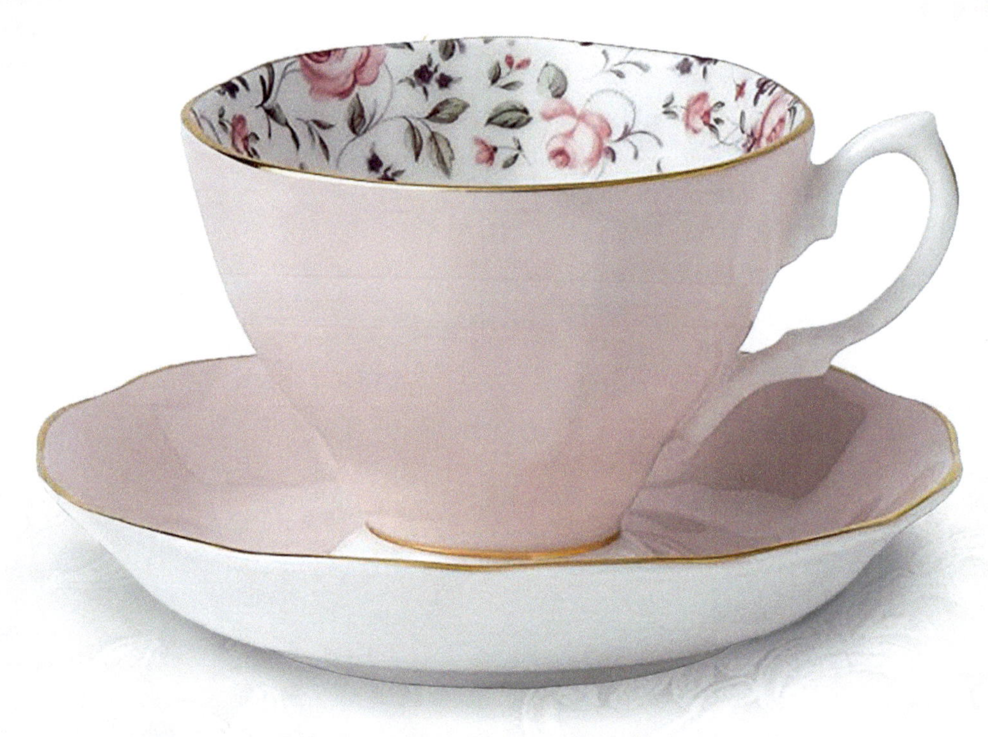

ROYAL ALBERT
ROSE CONFETTI

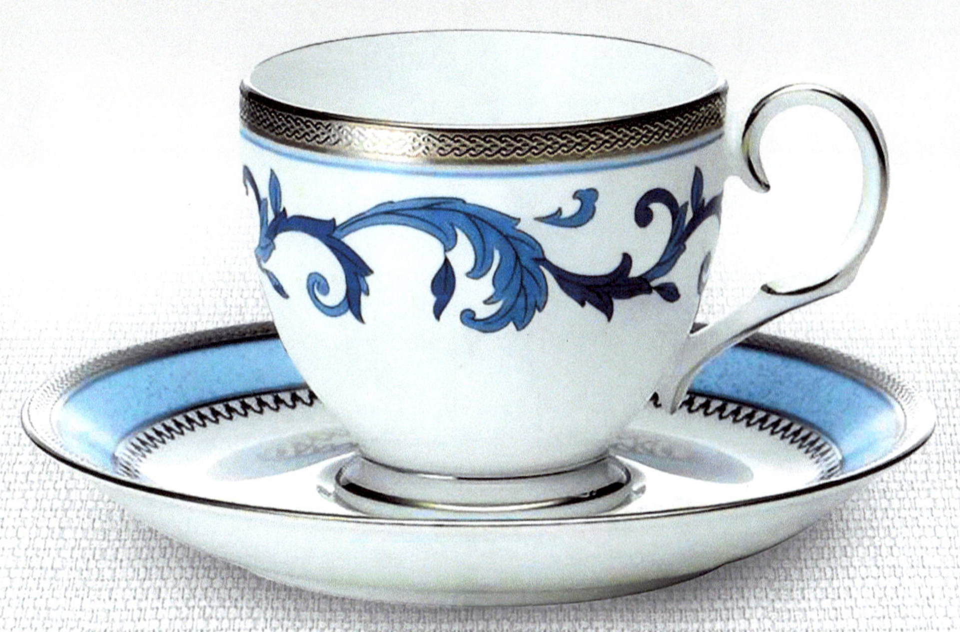


NORITAKE
SONNET IN BLUE

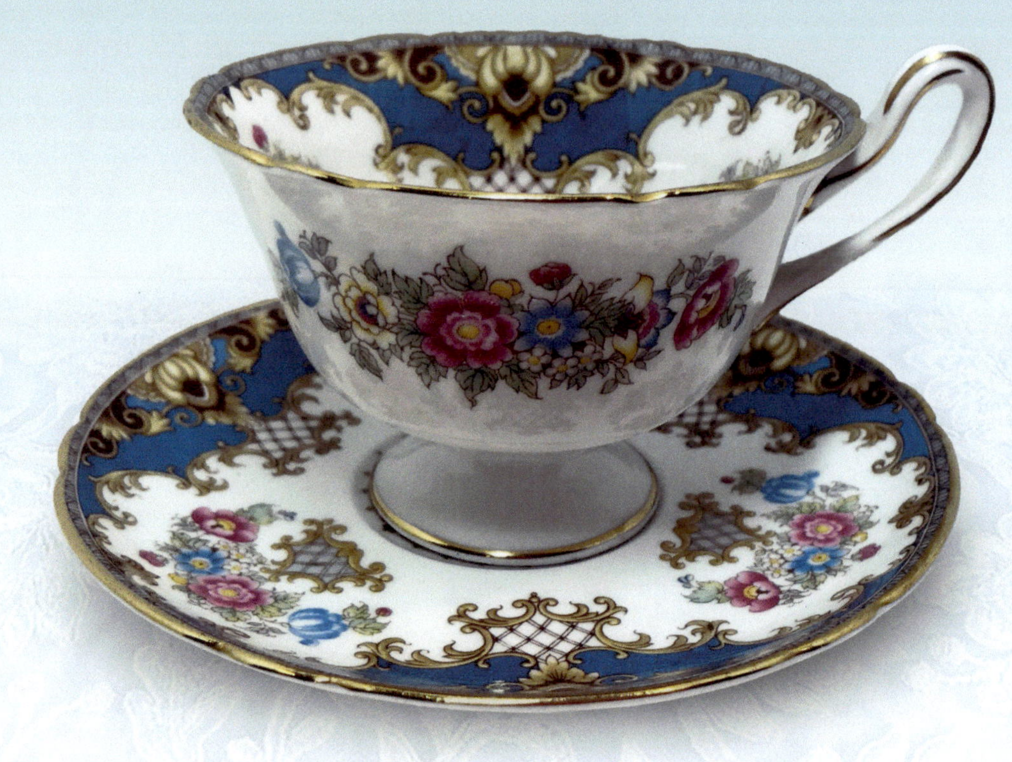

SHELLEY
SHERATON BLUE

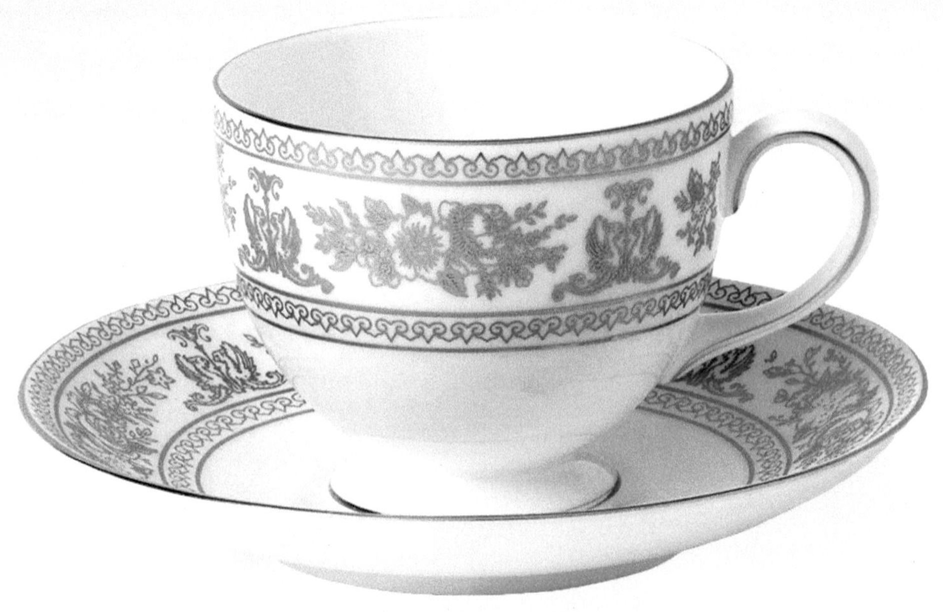

WEDGWOOD
COLUMBIA GOLD

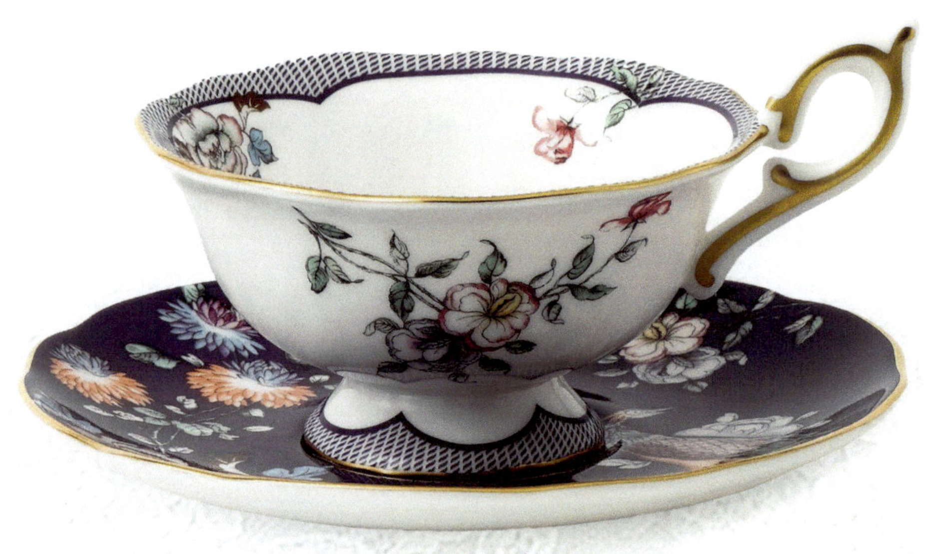

# WEDGWOOD

## WONDERLUST

## MIDNIGHT CRANE

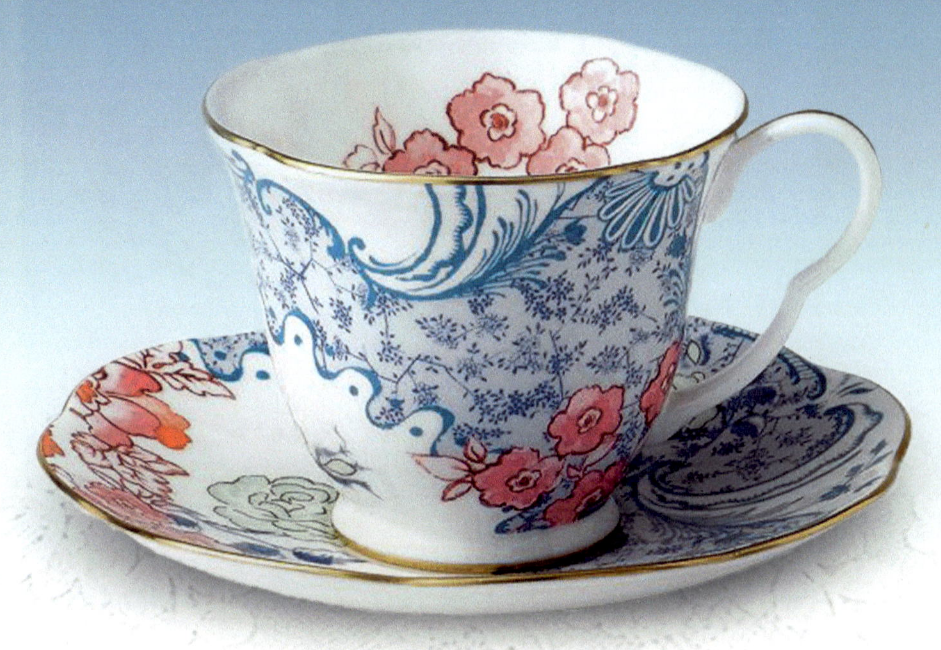

# WEDGEWOOD

## SPRING BLOSSOM

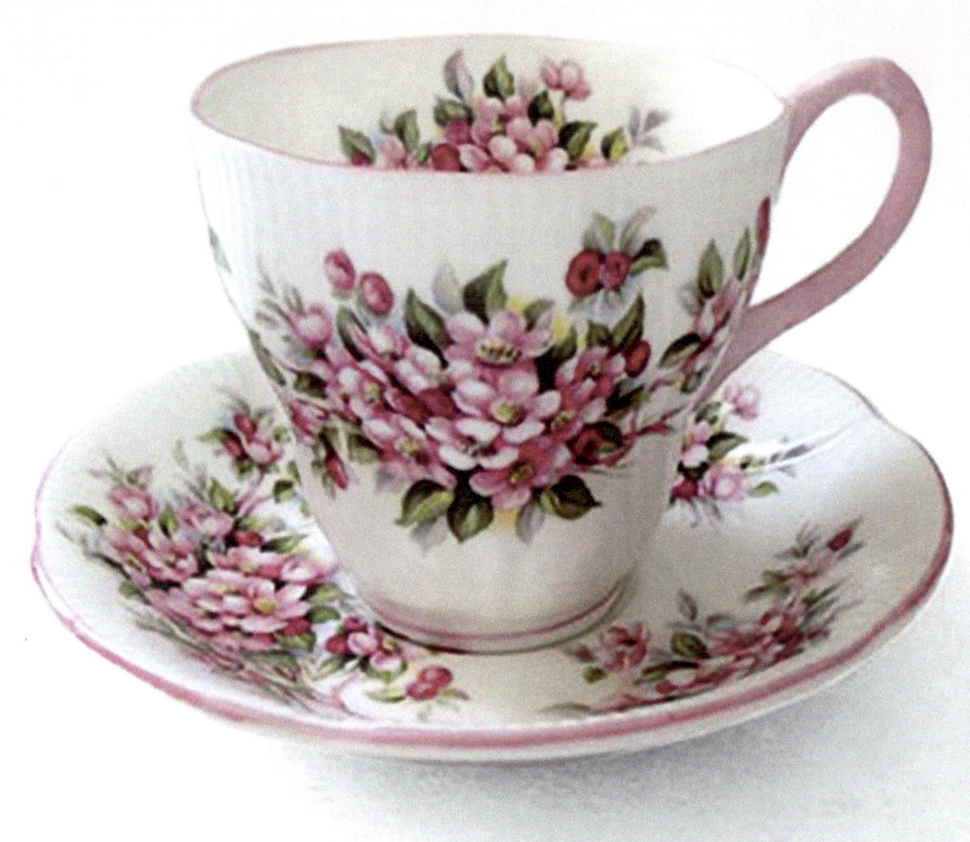

# ROYAL ALBERT

## APPLE BLOSSOM

### BLOSSOM TIME SERIES

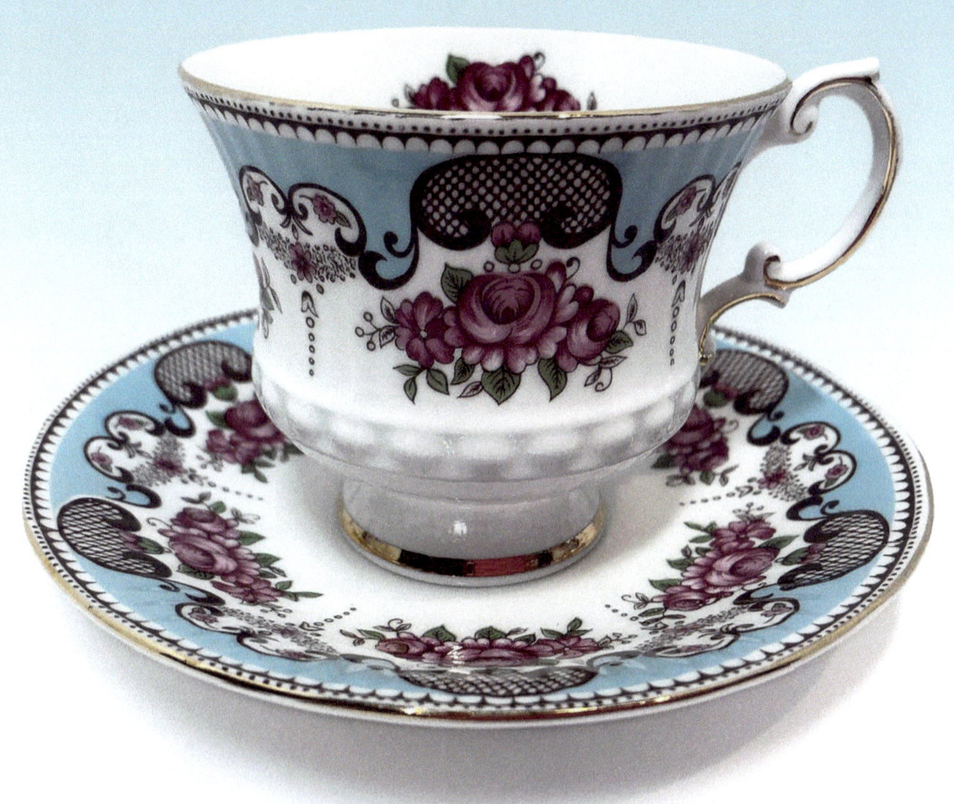

# ELIZABETHAN

## ASHBOURNE

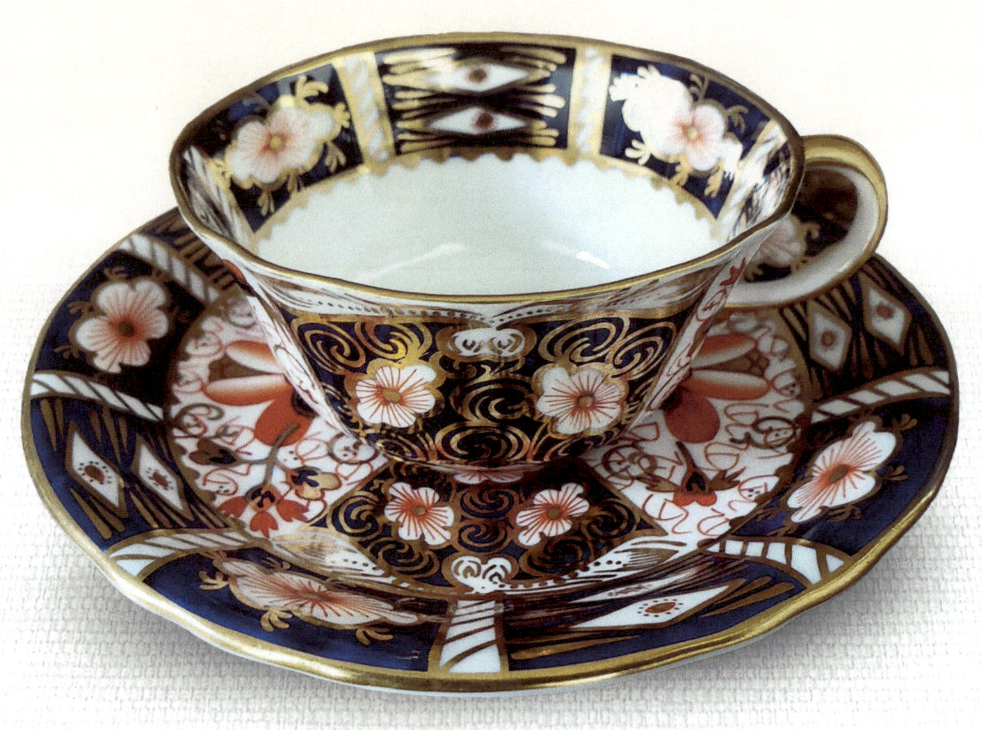


ROYAL CROWN DERBY

IMARI

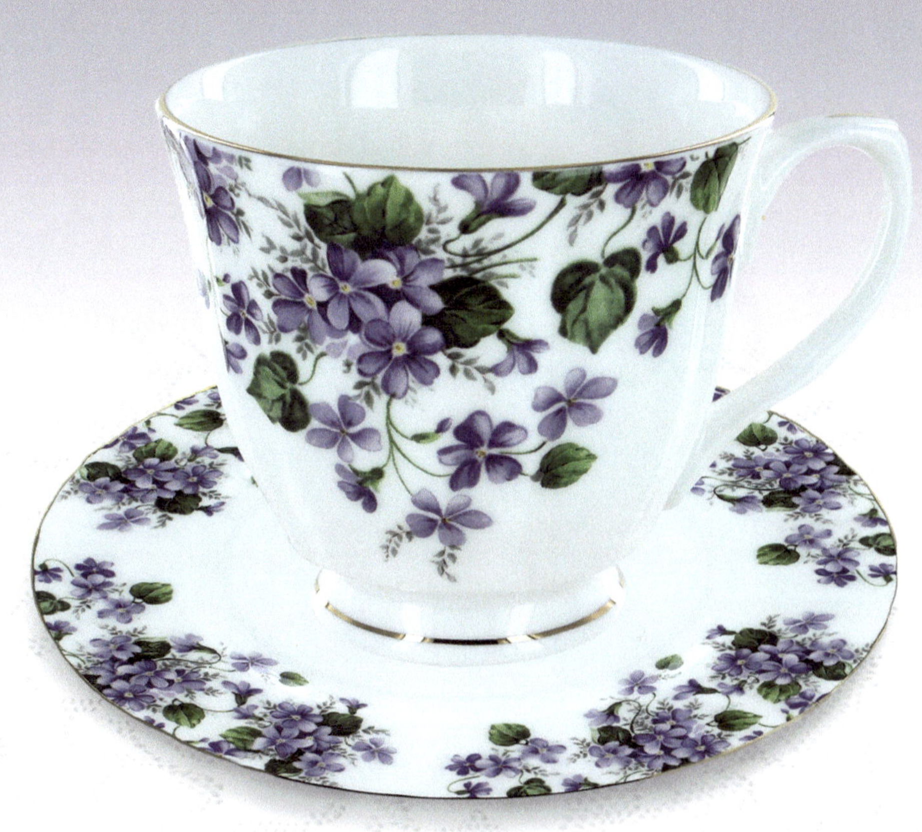

# GRACIE BONE CHINA
## VIOLETS

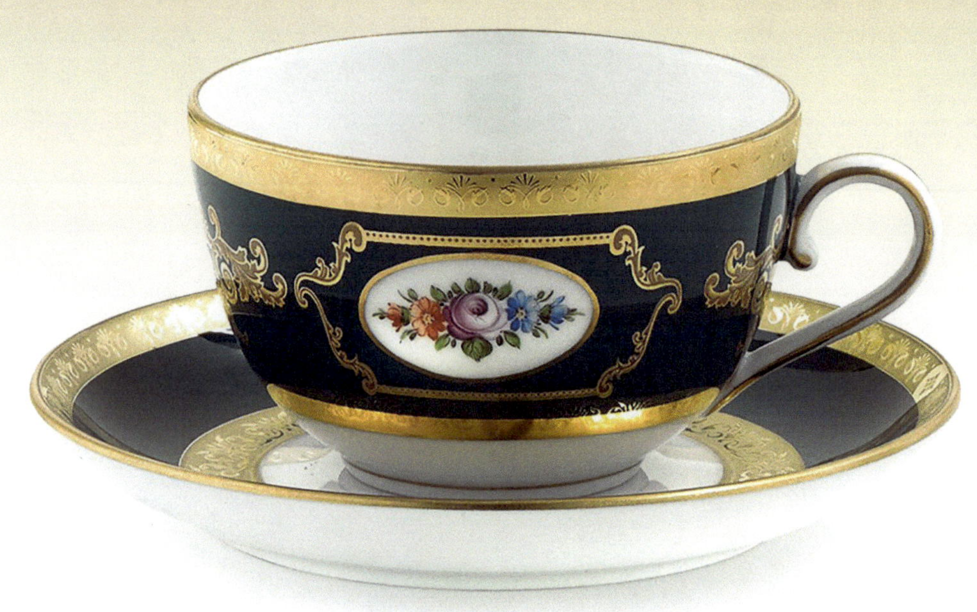

# HEREND

## SPLENDID

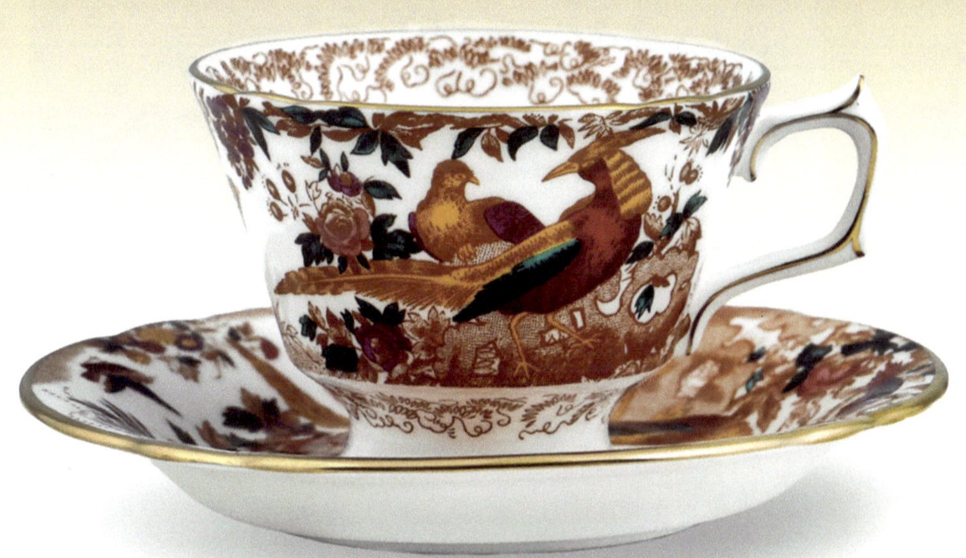

ROYAL CROWN DERBY

OLD AVESBURY

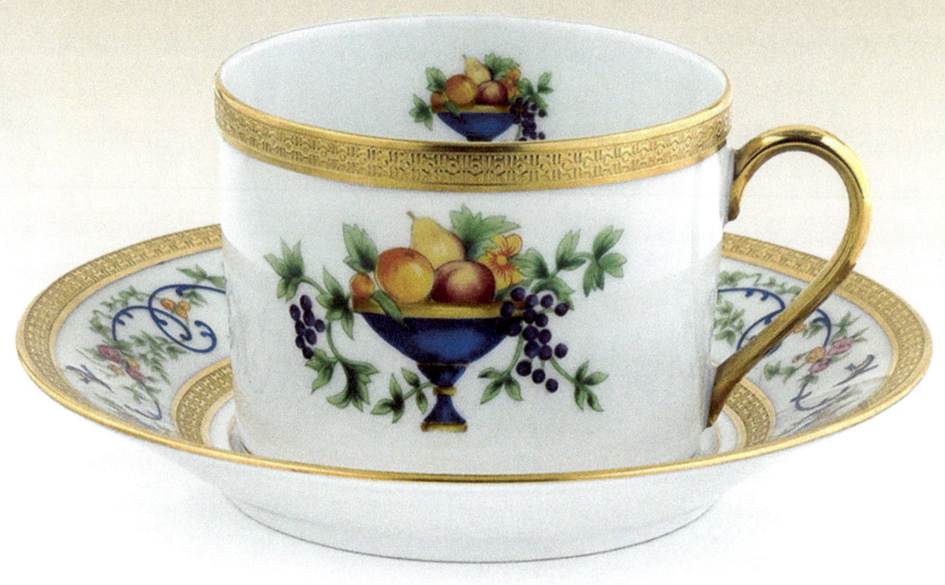


HAVILAND

VILLECROZE

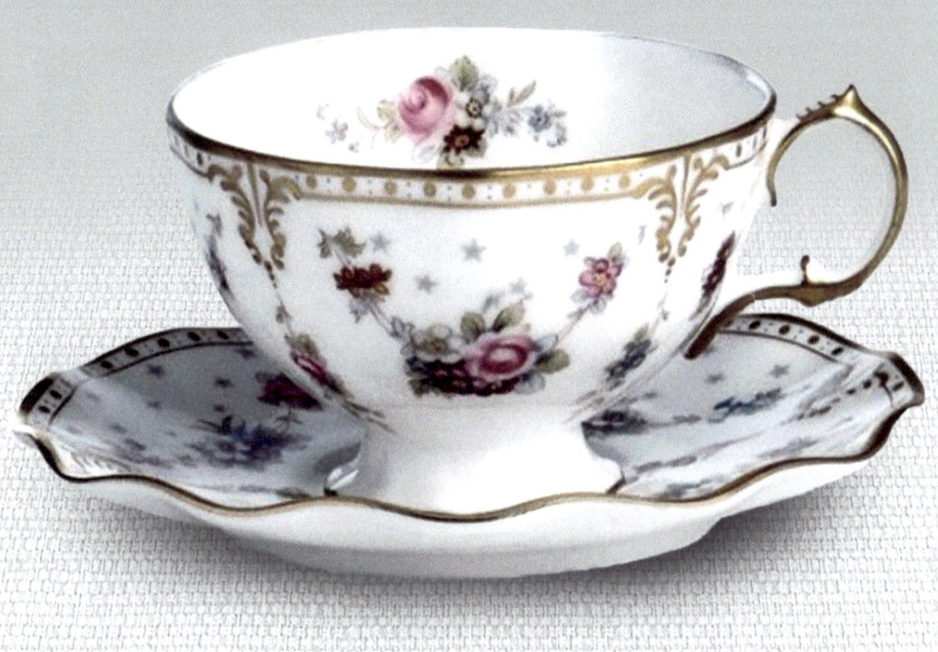


ROYAL CROWN DERBY

ROYAL ANTOINETTE

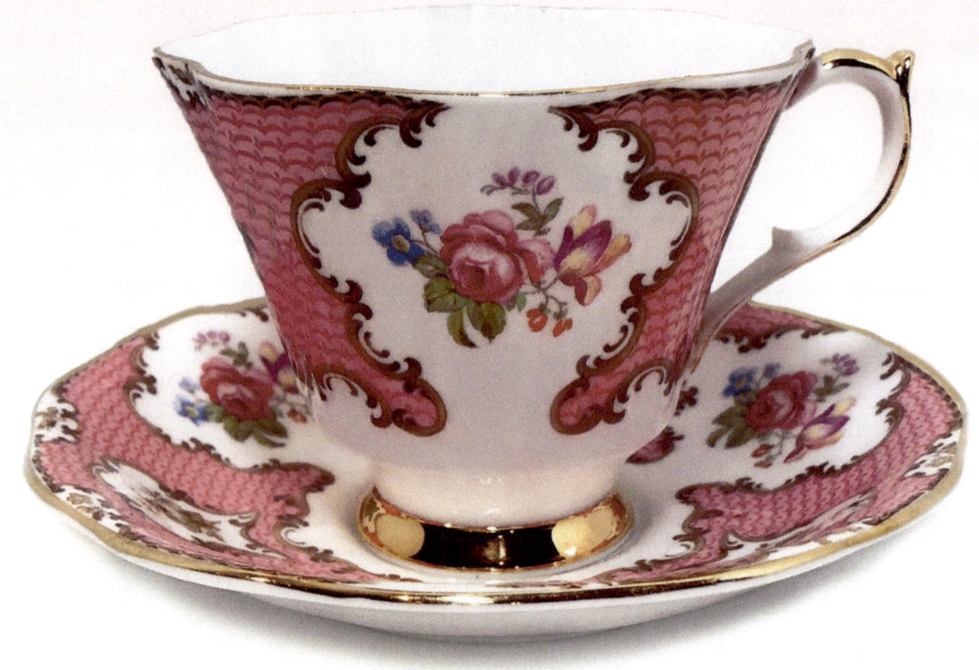

# QUEEN ANNE
## LADY ELEANOR

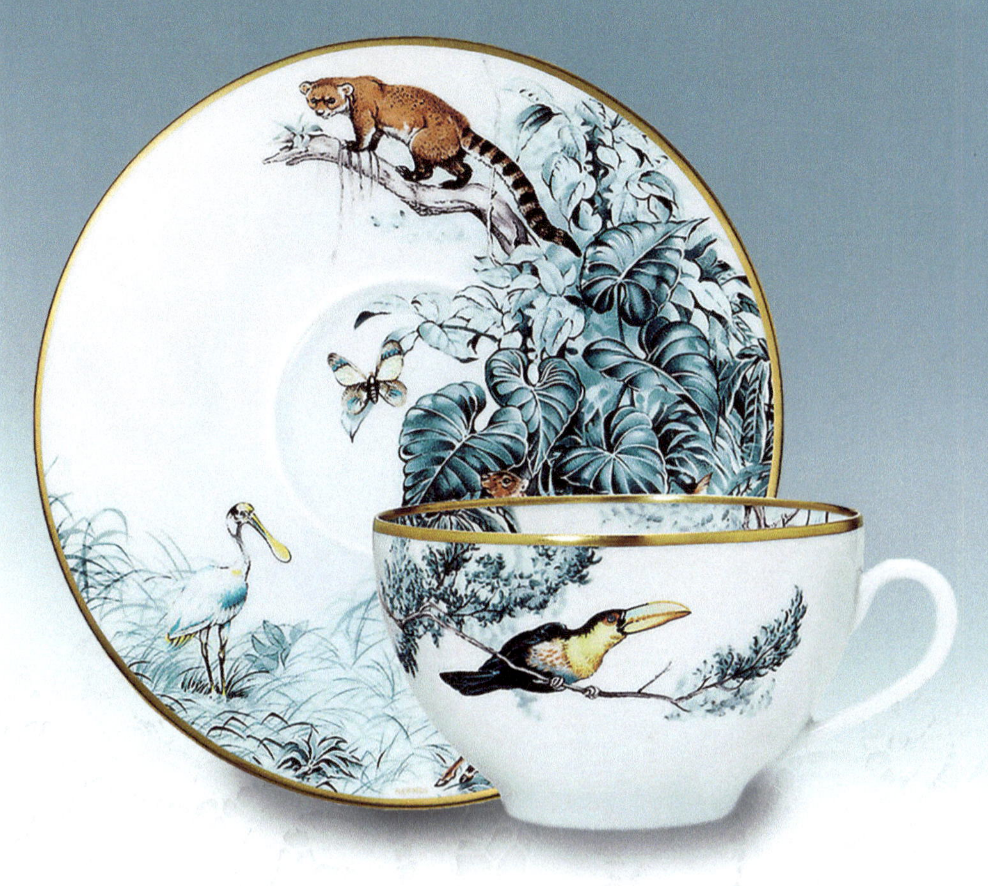

# HERMES

## CARNETS D'EQUATEUR

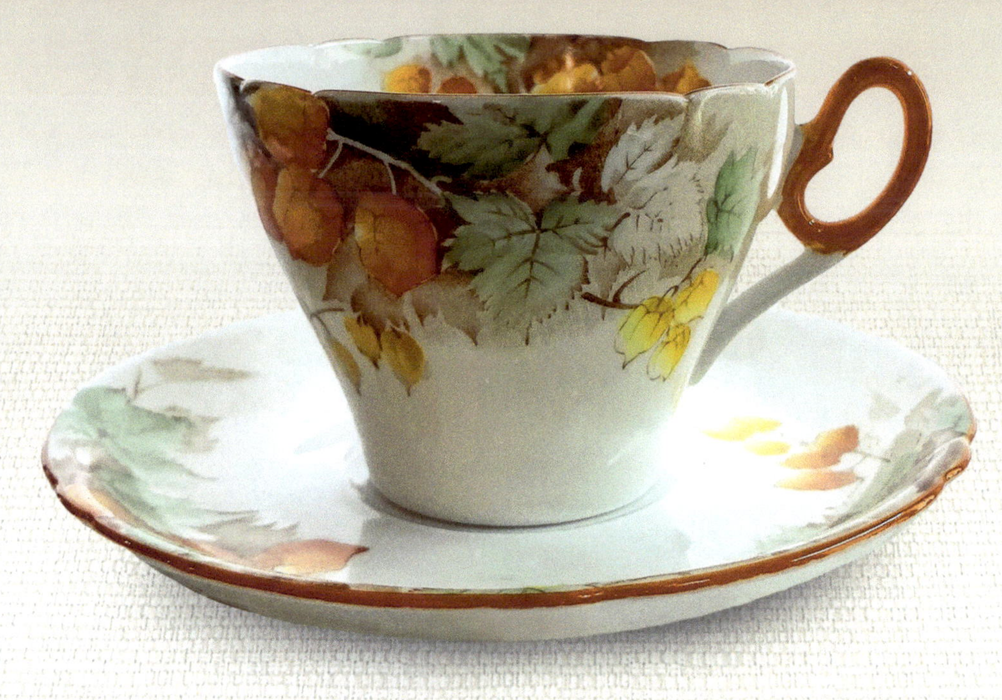


SHELLEY
OLD CAMBRIDGE
ORANGE WISTERIA

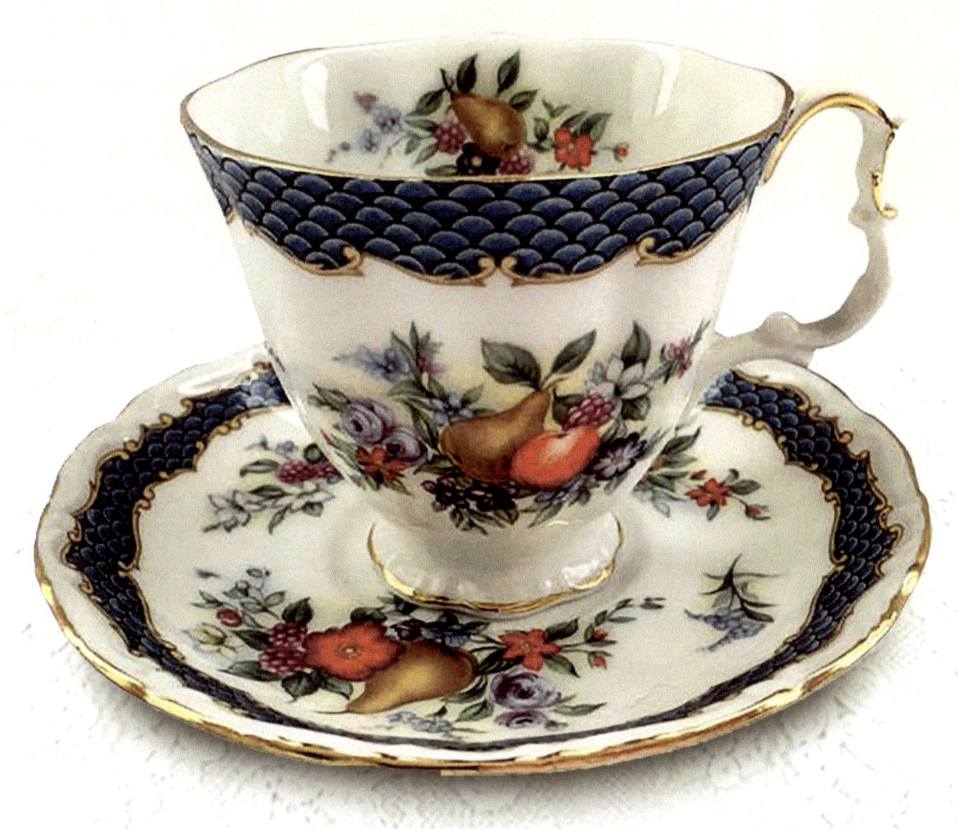


ROYAL ALBERT

BLUE LAGOON

IMPERIAL FRUIT SERIES

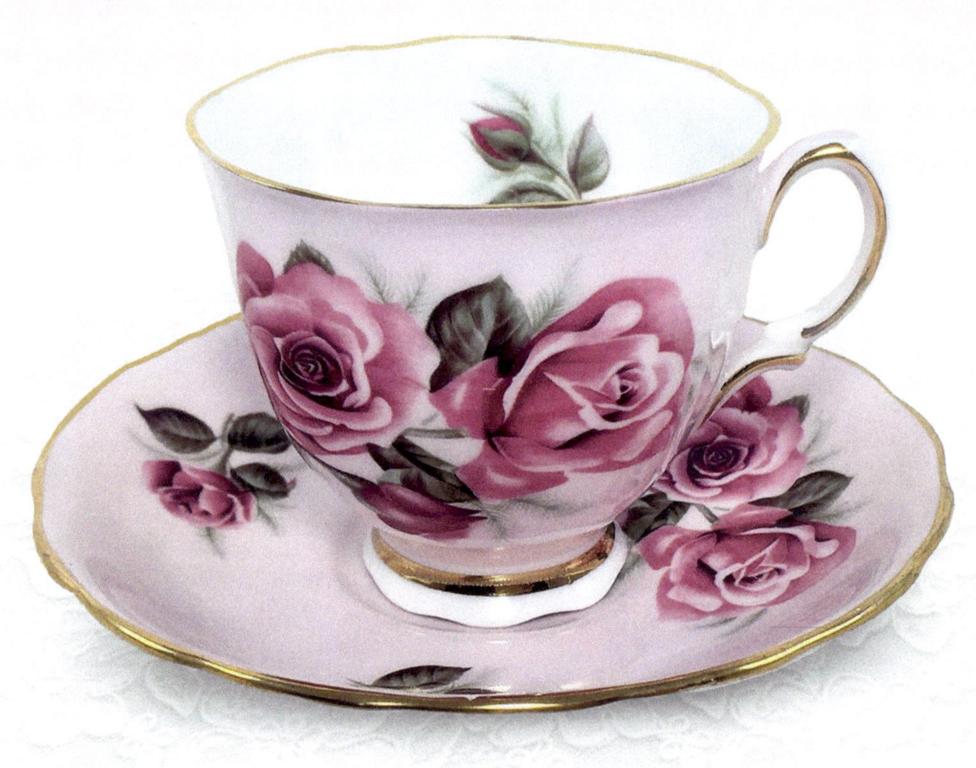

# COLCLOUGH

## PINK ROSES

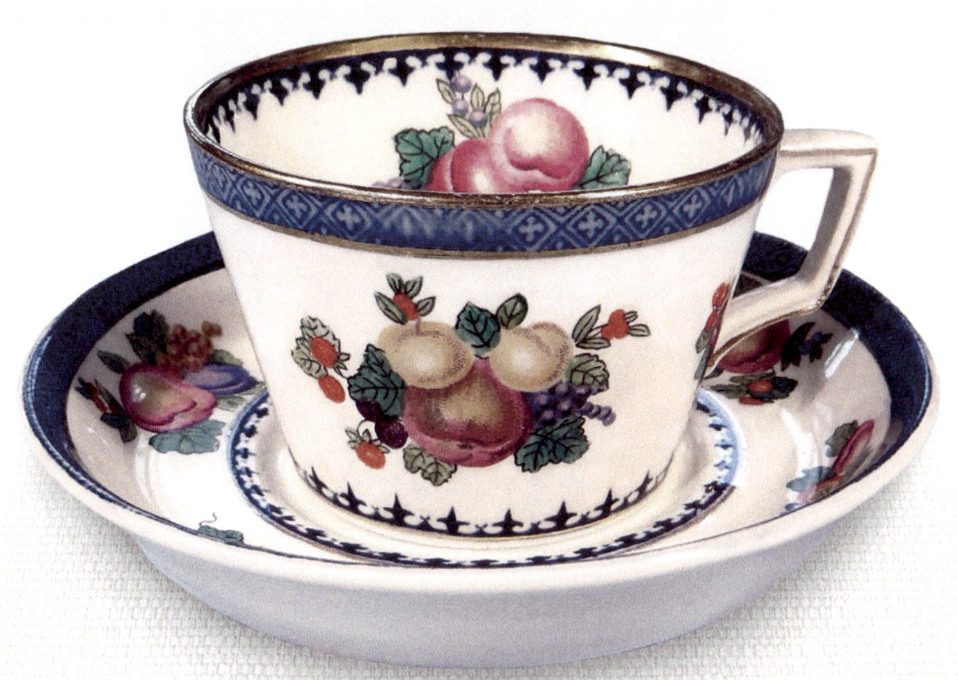

# BOOTHS

## SUMMER FRUITS

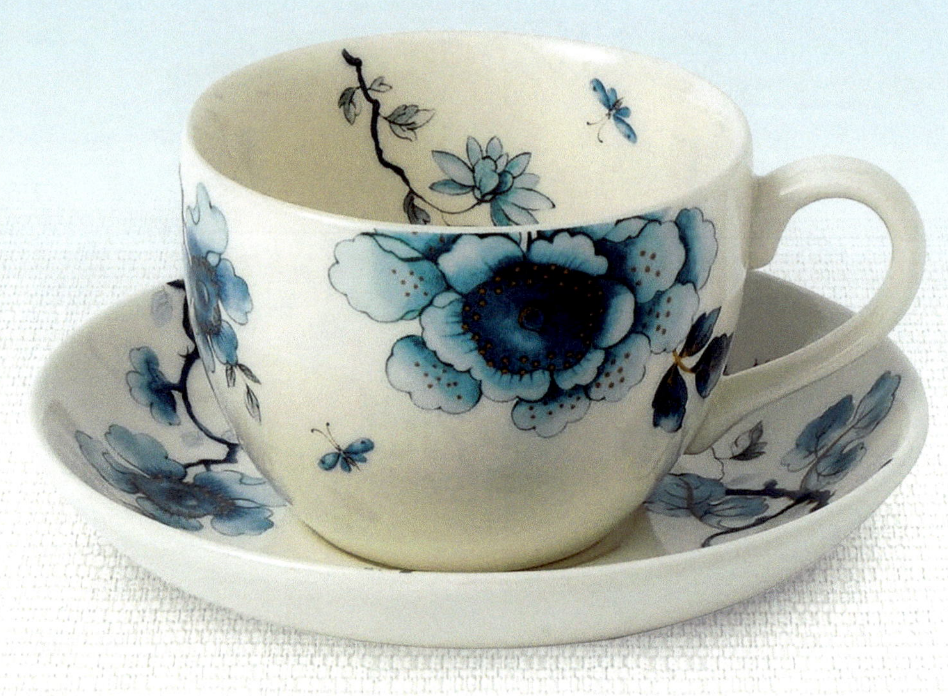

WEDGWOOD
BLUE BIRD

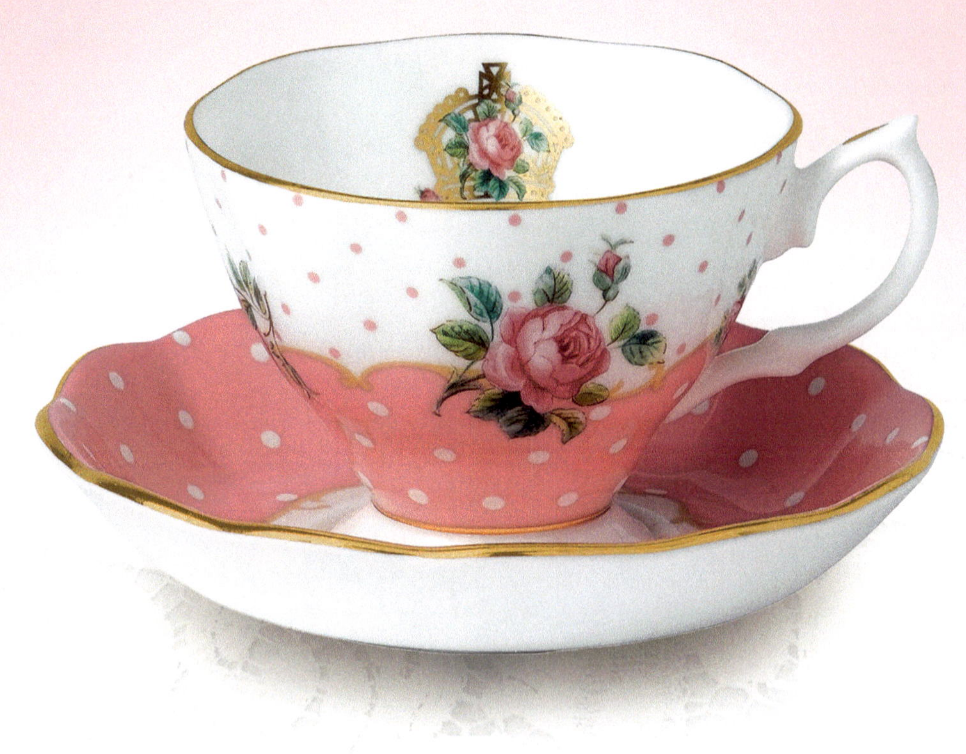

# ROYAL ALBERT
## CHEEKY PINK

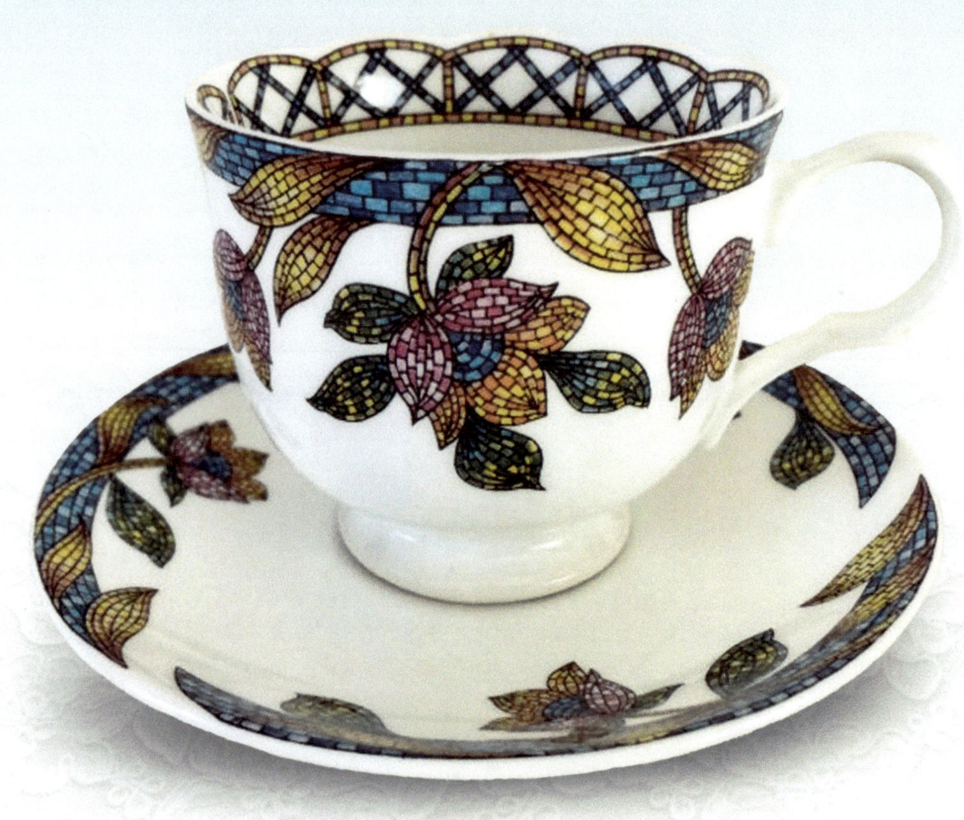

# SADLER

## PIAZZA MOSAIC

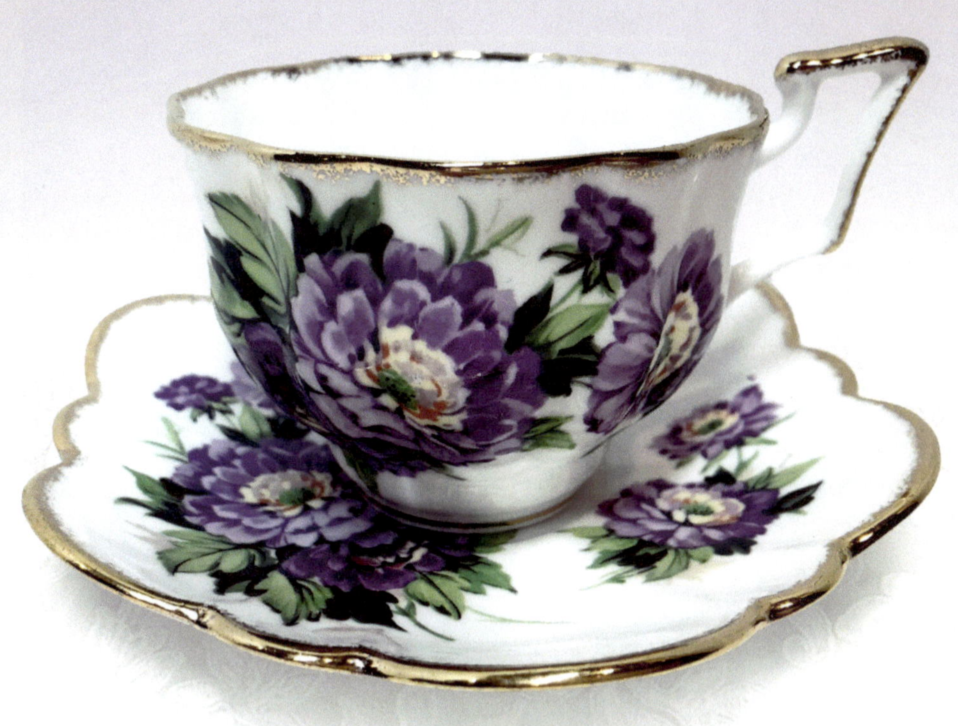


SALISBURY
EVENTIDE

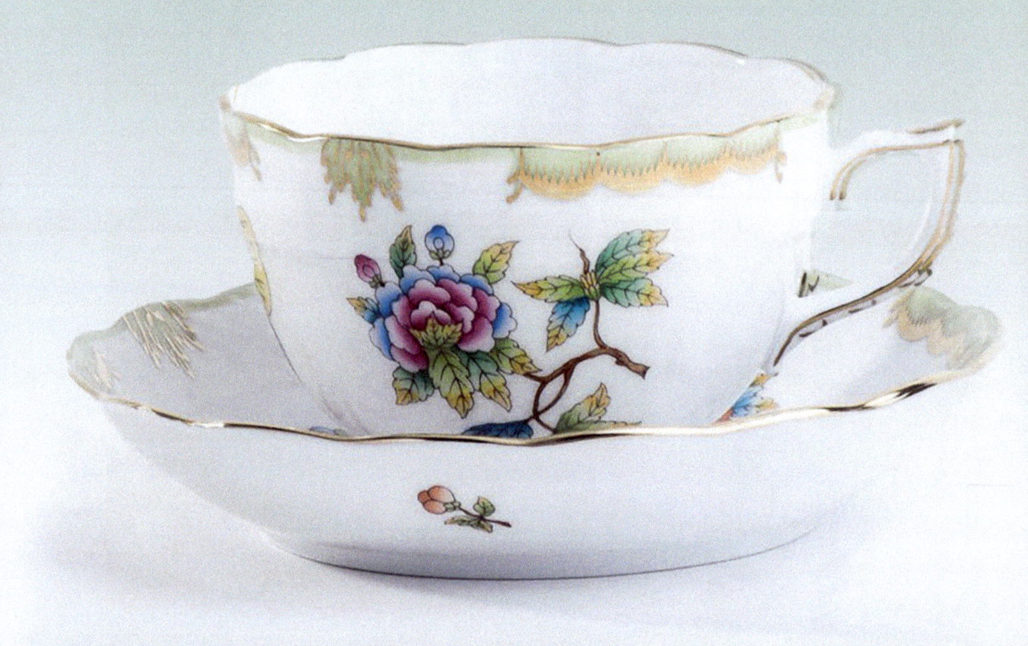

# HEREND

## QUEEN VICTORIA

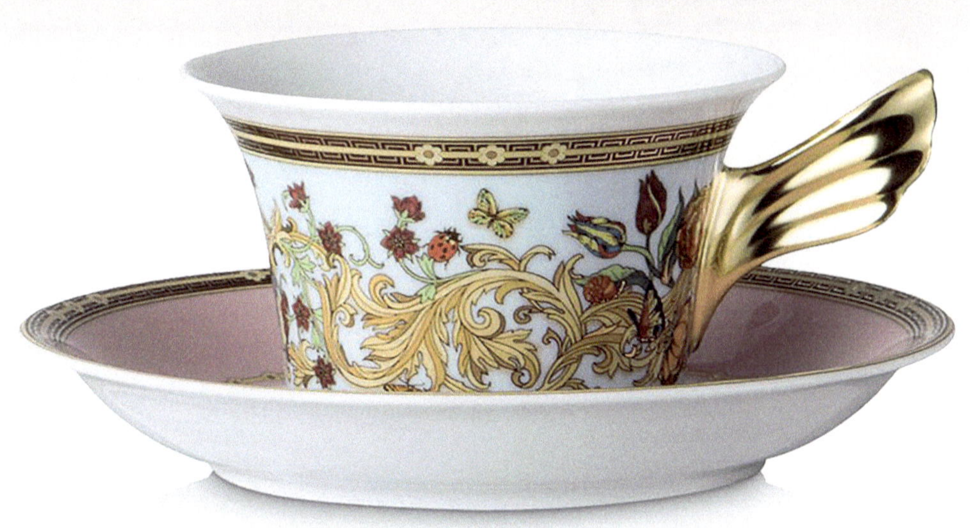

# VERSACE BY ROSENTHAL

## BUTTERFLY GARDEN

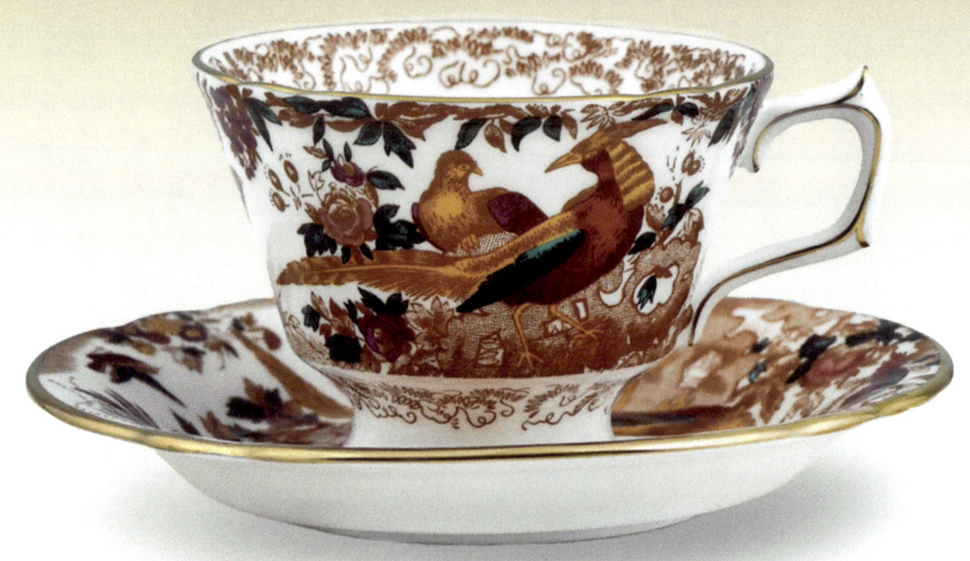

# ROYAL CROWN DERBY

## OLD AVESBURY

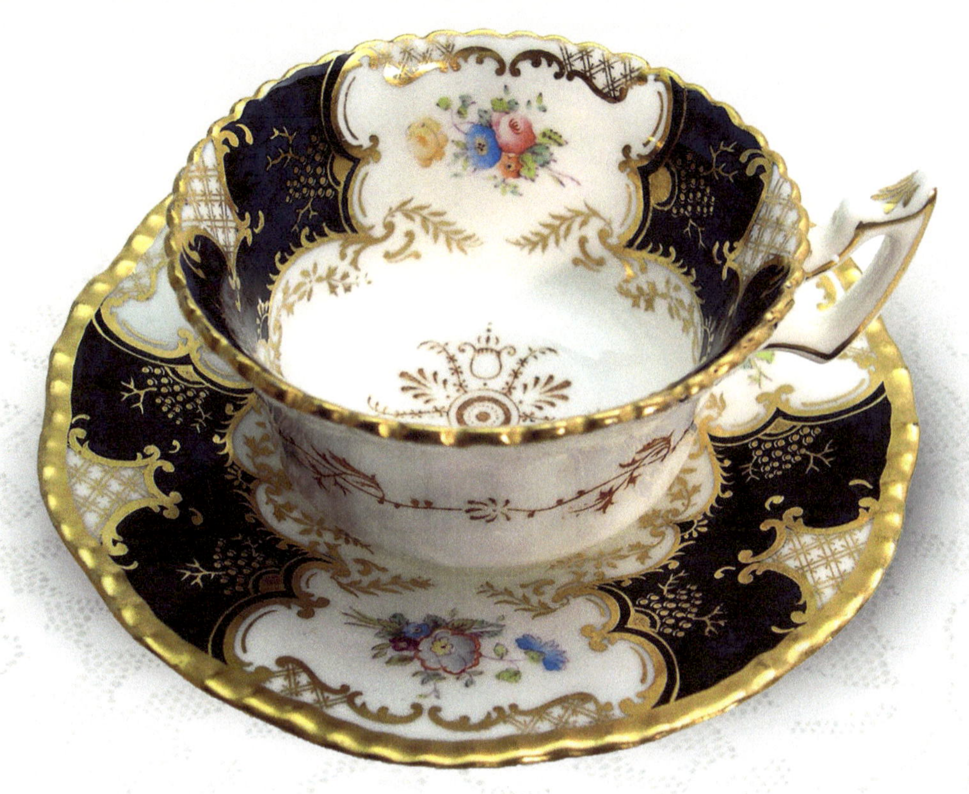

# COALPORT

## BATWING